D0280591

Top Tips for Fussy Eaters

Top Tips for Fussy Eaters

Gina Ford

Vermilion
LONDON

1 3 5 7 9 10 8 6 4 2

Published in 2010 by Vermilion, an imprint of Ebury Publishing
Ebury Publishing is a Random House Group company

The Random House Group Limited Reg. No. 954009
Addresses for companies within the Random House Group can be found at
www.rbooks.co.uk

A CIP catalogue record for this book is available from the British Library

The Random House Group Limited supports The Forest Stewardship
Council (FSC), the leading international forest certification organisation. All our
titles that are printed on Greenpeace approved FSC certified paper carry the FSC logo.
Our paper procurement policy can be found at www.rbooks.co.uk/environment

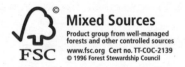

Mixed Sources

Product group from well-managed
forests and other controlled sources
www.fsc.org Cert no. TT-COC-2139
© 1996 Forest Stewardship Council

Printed and bound in Great Britain by CPI Mackays, Chatham, ME5 8TD

ISBN 9780091935153

To buy books by your favourite authors and register for offers, visit www.rbooks.co.uk

The information in this book has been compiled by way of general guidance in relation to the
specific subjects addressed, but is not a substitute and not to be relied on for medical, healthcare,
pharmaceutical or other professional advice on specific circumstances and in specific locations.
Please consult your GP before changing, stopping or starting any medical treatment. So far as the
author is aware the information given is correct and up to date as at February 2010. Practice, laws
and regulations all change, and the reader should obtain up-to-date professional advice on any such
issues. The author and publishers disclaim, as far as the law allows, any liability arising directly or
indirectly from the use, or misuse, of the information contained in this book.

Contents

Acknowledgements

Acknowledgements

I would like to thank to express my thanks and gratitude to the thousands of parents whom I have worked with or advised over the years. Their constant feedback, opinions and suggestions have been an enormous help in writing my books.

As always, I would also like to thank my publisher Fiona MacIntrye and editor Julia Kellaway for their constant encouragement and faith in my work, and Cindy Chan and the rest of the team at Vermilion for their careful work on this book. Special thanks are also owed to my agent Emma Kirby for her continued support and dedication.

I would also like to thank Registered Dietitian Fiona Hinton for her invaluable advice and expertise on various aspects of nutritional needs of children, and Kate Brian, the website editor of Contentedbaby.com, for her efforts in gathering information for the book. Thank you, too, to Yamini Franzini, Laura Simmons, Jane Waygood, Rory Jenkins and the rest of the team at Contentedbaby.com for their support while I was writing this book and their wonderful work on the website.

Finally, this book would not be here were it not for the thousands of readers who constantly provide me with inspiration and feedback. I am ever grateful for your huge support – thank you all and much love to you and your contented babies.

Introduction

Most children have some foods that they don't like or won't eat, and it is common for young children to go through a stage in their development when they are fussy about food. They may suddenly refuse to eat certain foods, demand ketchup with everything or insist that different foods aren't touching one another on their plates, but most of these phases will pass with time. However, fussy eating can sometimes become much more severe, with children limiting their diets to such an extent that every mealtime turns into a battleground and parents worrying that their child's nutritional requirements are not being met.

Fussy eating can start at any time between one and three years but it can be particularly bad if your toddler is drinking too much milk for his age. After three years, most children will begin to grow out of their fussy habits. Generally, if your child has been weaned on a variety of foods, fussy eating is less common, but even those who start out eating well can sometimes suddenly develop odd eating habits.

You know you have a fussy eater if you find that you are cooking the same thing every evening because your child refuses anything else; if you spend most of every mealtime arguing about food with your child; or are forever throwing away meals that you've spent hours preparing. It can seem that the more you try to persuade your child to eat at least one of the green things on his plate, the more stubborn he becomes in his refusal.

If your family mealtimes have become a battle, you may find that you get anxious and stressed before the start of every meal, worried about the arguments you expect to follow and concerned about what your child is going to agree to eat. I've met many parents who feel that their child is not eating enough, or not eating enough of the right foods, and difficult mealtimes can become set in a pattern that is hard to break.

I don't believe that feeding should ever become a source of anxiety for parents. Most common eating issues can be solved with some fairly simple practical advice, and I hope that this book will help you avoid some of the pitfalls that can lead to fussy eating and offer solutions to the difficulties that can arise. With the right approach, you will be able to help your child learn good eating habits which will keep him happy and healthy.

It is important to take action if food has become an issue for you and your child. A balanced diet is vital for young children as they are growing fast and their bodies are changing very rapidly. They need to eat a variety of foods to ensure they get all the essential nutrients that their bodies require. Your child should be eating foods from each of the four main food groups – protein, dairy, carbohydrate and fruit and vegetables – every day to ensure that he is getting the vitamins, minerals and trace elements that he needs. A child's nutrition can be linked to his intellectual and physical development later in life, and that's why it is so vital to develop good eating habits at an early age.

Eating a balanced diet is not just about getting the right fuel for your child's growing body, it is also about setting a pattern of healthy eating for the rest of his life. If you can encourage your child to try different foods, to eat well and to enjoy a varied diet, you will be laying down strong foundations for a good relationship with food for the future.

1
What are Healthy Eating Habits?

If you want to ensure your child has a healthy diet, it is important to start by understanding his nutritional requirements. Balance is the key, and children should be eating a variety of different foods, taking in each of the main food groups, to ensure that they get all the essential nutrients that their bodies need.

There are four main food groups – protein, dairy, carbohydrate and fruit and vegetables – and your child should be eating foods from each group every day. His needs will change as he grows, but it is important that you try to introduce him to a wide variety of different foods during the first few years of his life as this will help establish healthy eating habits for the future.

What your child needs

The first year

Breast or formula milk contains the nutrients that your baby needs for the first six months of his life. Solids are normally only introduced once your child reaches six months, when he can gradually move on to a variety of puréed and then mashed foods. By the end of the first year, he should be familiar with many types of vegetables, fruits, carbohydrates, dairy foods and protein, and will no longer need everything mashed or puréed. If you have managed to offer your child a wide range of different foods when he is still young, he is more likely to be willing to try new things as he gets older.

One and above

By the time your child is one, he will be following an adult eating pattern with three main meals a day. Some children are not keen to eat at breakfast time, but this is an important meal as it provides energy to start the day. Children who don't eat breakfast often get tired or bad-tempered later on. If your child eats a good breakfast and some protein with his lunch, this will give him the fuel he needs to keep him going throughout the day.

You should ensure that your child is getting what he needs from the four main food groups every day.

❖ **Protein** – your child needs a minimum of two portions of protein a day, depending on age and weight, from meat or meat alternatives. This can be meat, fish or pulses, such as lentils or beans. Avoid giving meats such as ham or bacon that are high in salt until your child is over two.

* **Dairy** – a one-year-old needs a minimum of 350ml (12oz) and a maximum of 500ml (17oz) of milk each day, and this can be follow-on formula or full-fat cow's milk. If your child is drinking too much milk, he may start to refuse to eat at mealtimes, therefore reducing his intake of solids which provide other essential nutrients. If he gets fussy about drinking milk, you can substitute some of the milk with yoghurt or fromage frais as they are both good sources of calcium. A 125g (4½oz) pot of yoghurt or 30g (1oz) of cheese is equivalent to 210ml (about 7oz) of milk.

Once your child is over the age of two, he will need around 350ml (12oz) of milk or other dairy products. He can now drink semi-skimmed cow's milk unless he is not gaining weight, in which case you may prefer to continue with full-fat milk.

* **Carbohydrate** – your child will need a minimum of three or four portions of carbohydrate each day. This can include bread, pasta, cereals, rice, potatoes, etc. Unrefined carbohydrates, which are the wholemeal and brown versions of

bread, pasta and rice, are better than the refined white versions which lose some of their nutrients in the refining process and are also converted to glucose more quickly.

❀ **Fruit and vegetables** – by the time he reaches a year, your child should be having at least five portions of fruit and vegetables every day. You can include raw or cooked, and canned or frozen, fruit and vegetables. Although people often worry that frozen or canned food is not as fresh, it is sometimes more nutritious because the fruit or vegetables have usually been picked and then prepared immediately, and therefore retain their nutrients. Fresh foods are sometimes kept in cold storage for a long time and may have lost some of their vitamin content.

Fruit and vegetable servings

It's not much use knowing how many portions of fruit and vegetables a child should be eating if you aren't sure what amount makes a portion. As a general guide, one portion of fruit or vegetables for a child under the age of six may be:

* One small apple, pear or banana, or half of a large one.
* Half a cup of grapes or berries.
* One small satsuma or tangerine.
* An apricot or kiwi fruit.
* One to two tablespoonfuls of vegetables.
* Half a bowl of salad.

Protein servings

The amount of protein a child needs is based on his age and his weight. Between one and three years of age it is recommended that children need around 16g (0.6oz) of protein a day, between four and six years this increases to around 24g (0.8oz) a day. There is about 6g (0.2oz) of protein in 25g (0.9oz) of lean meat or poultry, or in 35g (1.2oz) of white fish. Half a cup of beans, 180ml (6oz) of milk or 30g (1oz) of cheese also contain around 6g (0.2oz) of protein. Other foods high in protein would be an egg, half a cup of yoghurt or a tablespoon of peanut butter, each with around 4g (0.1oz).

Other foods, such as grain foods, also contain a smaller amount of protein. For example, a thin slice of bread, 100g (3½oz) of boiled rice, or 25g (0.9oz) of breakfast cereal each contain around 2g (0.1oz) of protein.

The recommended amounts are designed to meet the needs of almost all children of this weight and age. Registered dietitian Fiona Hinton advises that parents should not worry if some days children eat more, and some days children eat less. Many will not require quite as much as this, and most probably make up for it on other days anyway.

If you are following the recipes and menu planners in my books *The Gina Ford Baby and Toddler Cook Book*, *Feeding Made Easy* or *The Contented Little Baby Book of Weaning*, you can be reassured that they have been calculated to ensure that you child receives enough protein in his diet. For example, if your toddler eats a lunch recipe with around one to two ounces of animal protein in it, then something like pasta and a vegetable sauce or vegetable soup and bread will be more than sufficient for his tea. However, if for some reason he refuses lunch or only eats half of it, then giving him something like pasta with a cheese sauce or scrambled egg or beans on toast will more than make up for the protein he didn't have at lunchtime.

If you are introducing your child to a vegetarian diet, it is important to seek expert advice. Non-meat foods need to be combined correctly to provide your child with a complete source of protein. Examples of food combinations for vegetarians that provide this are beans mixed with rice, wheat, corn, oats or barley, breakfast cereal with milk, or pasta with cheese. However, you should discuss with your health visitor or GP before starting your child on a vegetarian diet.

Don't worry if your child sometimes eats far more or far less than the recommended amount. As long as he is growing and developing healthily and eating a variety of foods from all the main food groups, he is likely to be getting the protein he needs.

Vitamins and minerals

Your child needs essential vitamins and minerals in order to grow and flourish, but it would be a full-time task to monitor his diet to check his daily intake of every one of the vitamins and minerals he needs. If your child is eating a balanced diet from each of the main food groups, he is unlikely to be lacking in any essential vitamins and minerals. It is generally only when a child refuses to eat from certain food groups that problems arise. Some essential vitamins and minerals include:

✿ **Calcium** – found in milk and dairy products. It ensures the development of healthy bones and teeth. You can also find calcium in pulses, leafy green vegetables, dried fruit, nuts, seeds and canned fish.

* **Iron** – found in red meat, offal and oily fish. One study found that more than 10 per cent of toddlers were deficient in iron, and children who don't have enough iron can become anaemic. Iron can also be found in eggs (which should be cooked until both the yolk and white are solid), beans and lentils, dried fruit, broccoli and leafy green vegetables, as well as some breakfast cereals and baby foods that are fortified with iron.

   Be careful about offering too much liver to a toddler who is deficient in iron, as liver foods should only be consumed once a week by young children. Liver contains high levels of vitamin A, and large amounts of this can be dangerous to young children.

* **Vitamin C** – found in fruits (especially citrus fruit and juice), kiwi fruit, strawberries, green vegetables and tomatoes. It is important to eat foods containing vitamin C regularly as the body can't store it. Vitamin C helps with the growth and repair of body cells and also helps fight infection.

* **Vitamin D** – obtained from sunlight, but in countries where

there is very little exposure to the sun, it can be sourced from food. It is found in margarine, butter, evaporated milk, eggs, oily fish and liver.

Fat

As adults, we tend to think of fat as unhealthy and although too much fat is bad for us, children need fat as they are growing and developing rapidly. Fat has the highest energy content per gram of any food we consume.

Fats also contain vitamins A, D, E and K. Generally, vegetable fats (such as vegetable oils) are healthier than those derived from animals (such as butter or lard) with the exception of fish fat which has many benefits. Polyunsaturated fats, found in nuts, seeds, fish and vegetable oils, are healthier than the saturated fats found in meat and coconut or palm oils.

If your child is underweight, you can help give him the fuel his body needs by melting butter over vegetables or frying foods, although these are things you would try to avoid as an adult. If you have any worries about your child's weight, you should always contact your health visitor or GP.

Essential fatty acids – Omega-3 and Omega-6

* **Omega-3 fats** – children's bodies need these polyunsaturated fats in order to grow and develop properly. They are found in oily fish (such as salmon, mackerel and fresh tuna) and in certain oils (such as flaxseed or walnut oil), as well as in some soy-based foods such as tofu. You should try to include at least one portion of oily fish in your child's diet each week.

* **Omega-6 fats** – also essential to development, but these are found more widely in our daily diet in food such as vegetable oils, margarine, seeds and nuts.

Salt and sugar

Salt and sugar are both added to many processed foods to give flavour. If your child eats too many processed foods, he may become accustomed to these flavours in all his food.

* Salt can be really dangerous for babies, and may lead to high blood pressure, strokes and heart disease later in life.

* Children of 1–2 years should not have more than 2g of salt a day and children of 4–6 years can have a maximum of 3g of salt a day.

* Don't add salt to meals you make for the whole family. Make the dish and separate your child's portion before salting your own.

* Try to avoid giving sugary drinks and never give a baby sweet drinks from a bottle, especially at bedtime, as this can lead to dental decay.

- Sugar is often added to processed foods under a different name, so you may see sucrose, glucose, fructose, maltose or corn syrup on the ingredients label.

- Maltodextrins are partially broken-down sugars that are found in some processed baby foods. They have no nutritional benefits and are not found naturally in foods. Avoid giving baby foods containing maltodextrins.

- Try to check all food labels for amounts of salt and sugar, particularly in bread, soups and beans.

Case study: Anya, aged 2 years and 10 months
Problem: Fantastic feeder to fussy eater
Cause: Over-compensating for likes and dislikes

Sophie went back to work when her daughter, Anya, was six months old and a nanny took over during the day. Anya had already been weaned and took really well to solids. She would take a whole range of foods and her favourites were spinach and potato, liver, shepherd's pie and cod with sweet potato. Anya continued to eat well and with great enthusiasm under the care of the nanny.

Then Sophie decided to give up work when Anya was 20 months old. The nanny left and Anya's eating habits seemed to change overnight. To Sophie's surprise, in the first couple of weeks when she had sole care of her daughter, Anya began to refuse some of her meals and the problem became more pronounced until Anya began constantly to refuse her meals. Sophie responded by becoming increasingly anxious. The nanny had been hugely competent, and Sophie felt that her daughter must be reacting to the change in routine. Sophie tried to entice Anya to eat *and would offer her alternatives if one of the favourite foods was rejected, but within a fortnight of the nanny's departure Sophie had resorted to giving the few foods Anya was now prepared to eat – yoghurt and grated cheese. Mealtimes became increasingly upsetting, with Anya pushing foods onto the floor and Sophie almost crying with frustration.*

Within two months it had reached a stage where Anya was eating only Weetabix with banana, jam sandwiches, biscuits, chocolate and ice cream. Sophie did occasionally try to withdraw biscuits between meals, but Anya would cry and scream until Sophie gave in. Anya would not be hungry at mealtimes but would be hungry again later and demand more sweet things. Sophie couldn't get herself out of the habit of giving in to Anya's demands for biscuits and chocolates, and at this point she rang me for advice.

When I spoke to Sophie I said that it was of the utmost importance to get rid of all biscuits, sweets and ice cream from the house and to decide firmly that there must be no eating between meals. We prepared a menu plan for the next seven days and I told Sophie that if Anya cried and screamed for biscuits and sweets when she was given her meals, she was to walk away from her. She must not get into a conversation about food.

Sophie started the plan at the weekend so that her husband could support her. I suggested that they offer Anya a selection of fruits and yoghurt at breakfast instead of the usual Weetabix and banana to encourage her appetite for lunch. Lunch was always her worst meal, where she played up the most, refusing all forms of protein for the last five months. I suggested that Sophie shouldn't burden Anya with huge platefuls of food, but put small amounts, including some vegetables, on the plate. I explained that we should save the foods that we knew Anya would eat until teatime. We did not want her final meal of the day before bedtime to become a battle.

Sophie recognised with hindsight that her concern about her daughter missing the nanny had meant she had reacted too quickly to Anya's altered feeding habits. We both agreed that Anya, a bright little girl, had rapidly established that fussy eating was rewarded by her mother's undivided attention. The more Sophie responded, the more the pattern was set. Sugary snacks between meals ruined Anya's appetite and made it even less likely that she would eat wholesome food.

Reversing these patterns was going to be challenging. Anya had awful tantrums during the first three days and her sleep was affected. It was very upsetting for her parents. However, Sophie and her husband persevered and, to their delight, by the fourth morning Anya ate her fruit and yoghurt within eight minutes. At lunchtime, within 20 minutes, she happily ate fish fingers and peas with baby new potatoes. The pattern was broken.

Gradually, over the next few days, they reintroduced cereal and toast at breakfast time. Once they became confident that her lunchtime appetite had returned, they were able to increase her breakfast.

I encouraged her parents to give her nutritious finger foods at lunchtime. By doing this, Anya was able to feed herself, and while she was no longer in a position to choose her meals, she did have a level of control that pacified her. In addition, I told Sophie to praise her when she ate, but to ignore her if the food was either rejected or thrown from the high chair, and end the meal. Within the first week, Anya's diet had improved enormously. She was eating a very good breakfast, including porridge, toast fingers and cut-up fruit. Her lunch had the appropriate balance of nutritious food. By the second week, she was happily attempting to feed herself most of the meal using her fingers, and she was also allowing her mother to help. On the increasingly rare occasions when food was refused, Sophie responded by making no fuss, but offering no alternatives. Her daughter's stamina was improved, she no longer needed or expected sugary snacks between meals, and on the occasions when they were out the only snacks she was allowed were healthy ones in moderation – fruit, raisins and raw vegetables.

Toddlers are very sensitive to the response their behaviour generates. While Anya's response was *extreme, it was clearly motivated by her discovery that she could get her mother's attention by not eating. Her mother's lack of confidence in herself meant that she over-compensated for her daughter's fussy eating. Fortunately, they both re-established good feeding patterns, which they have been able to maintain to this day.*

Family influences

The way you eat as a family will shape your child's eating habits. If you tend to graze rather than have proper meals, eat in front of the TV or snack on the go, your child will follow these patterns. If you sit at the table for meals and eat together as a family, this will help establish your child's good habits for the future. What you eat will also make a difference – your child is not going to choose to eat lots of vegetables if he never sees you eating any. If you set a good example by eating healthily yourself, your child is far more likely to follow.

* Always try to make time for family meals if you possibly can. Watching you will help your child establish good table manners and will encourage him to enjoy eating healthily.

* Try not to worry if your child isn't hungry at one meal. Never force him to eat, or offer snacks as an alternative. He will probably make up for it at the next meal, or the next day. If you do become worried, keep a detailed food diary for one week of all food and drink consumed with exact times and amounts. Then make an appointment with your health visitor and they can discuss your concerns.

* Encourage your child to feed himself as much as he can during his second year. You do have to accept that it will be messy for a while.

- You can introduce your child to his own spoon, and also a knife and fork, between the ages of two and three. You can buy inexpensive children's cutlery which is designed to appeal to youngsters. Using these, he should manage to eat most of his meals without any assistance.

- Only encourage your child to use his fingers to eat if he is eating finger foods.

- From the age of four, you may want to buy some inexpensive china crockery for your child.

- You may want to continue using a bib if your child doesn't object as he will continue to get messy at mealtimes until he is used to feeding himself.

- Your child will learn good table manners if he is allowed to eat with adults in a relaxed environment.

- Some toddlers tend to hold their cutlery and beaker in their hands throughout the meal. Try to encourage them to put them down while they are chewing their food.

- Encourage your child to sit properly at the table, and praise him for sitting well with his elbows off the table and for saying please and thank you.

- If your child is constantly climbing down from the table before the meal is finished, you will need to be firm. Make it clear that once he leaves the table, he cannot come back to eat more food or for pudding.

- Your child may be more likely to get down from the table if he is free from a high chair or harness for the first time as he will be enjoying the freedom.

- Children are sometimes uncomfortable on adult chairs, and this can make them more inclined to get down from the table. Buying a booster seat or a special chair designed for young children may be helpful.

The key to ensuring your child has a healthy diet is to include a variety of foods from each of the main groups, and to make sure that he eats a fairly balanced diet. Many children develop fussy habits about certain foods at certain times so try not to worry too much about what he eats at each meal, or even each day, but make sure that over a few days he is getting all of the foods that he needs.

2

How to Prevent Fussy Eating Habits as Your Child Develops

Many toddlers and young children will get fussy about their food at some stage, and even those who have eaten well previously may suddenly decide that they don't like certain foods or start refusing to try new things. This isn't a huge problem as long as your child still has a balanced diet, and most will grow out of any minor fussy eating problems after a while. However, you can make all the difference to your child's eating habits by setting a good pattern at the very start, and by avoiding some of the common pitfalls that can lead to fussy eating. Sometimes an eating issue is exacerbated when parents start to worry about their child and offer alternative snacks if they don't eat meals. It is possible to avoid many common fussy eating issues if you establish good eating habits from an early age.

Laying the foundations for good eating habits

If your baby experiences a variety of different foods from a young age and learns to enjoy them, you are less likely to have problems with fussy eating when he gets older. During the latter part of the first year, if you have not already started, you can be more adventurous with your toddler's food, adding different spices and flavourings. You can also try offering him a taste of your meal when you eat out in restaurants to widen his experience of multicultural foods.

The second year

During the second year, children's appetites usually decrease considerably as their growth rate slows and they need fewer calories. At this age, children often seem to eat huge amounts of food one day, and then very little the next. Some parents get terribly worried about this, but it is perfectly normal. It is the overall intake of food over several days that is important, and keeping a food diary is often a good way of reassuring yourself that your child is getting what he needs.

* Make sure that you are aware of the main food groups (protein, dairy, carbohydrate and fruit and vegetables – see page 15), and of the quantities of each that your child should be eating. This will ensure his nutritional needs are met.

* If your toddler doesn't seem particularly hungry, don't force-feed him or insist that he eats when he doesn't want to. Sometimes building up this kind of anxiety around food can

lead to fussiness later on. Constant pressure on a child to eat can turn mealtimes into a battle of wills and establish a pattern which is hard to break.

* Encourage your child to drink milk from a beaker or cup during his second year, if he has not already started to do so. Your child can drink more quickly from a bottle and if you let him continue to drink from it he may fill up on milk, become fussier at mealtimes and even refuse to eat at some meals. To avoid this happening it is important that he always drinks from a cup and that the bottle is abandoned completely.

* Solids should become your child's main source of nutrition during this year, but milk still plays an important role in a balanced diet. A child of this age can be given full-fat cow's milk and should be drinking a minimum of 350ml (12oz) and a maximum of 500ml (17oz) a day. If your child is getting fussy about milk, you can offer yoghurt or extra cheese to boost his dairy intake.

* Don't get into the habit of bribing your child to eat his meals with the option of an unhealthy pudding or sweet if he finishes his main course. This could lead to mealtimes becoming a battle of wills with your child insisting on a sweet before he will eat his main course.

* If you schedule your meals at regular times and stick to them, this will help maintain healthy eating habits. Toddlers can get overtired very quickly as they use up a lot of energy, and need to eat regularly. Breakfast should be over by 8am, so that your child will be ready for lunch at around midday and tea at around 5pm.

* Your child will need snacks and drinks between meals, but schedule them so that they are not too close to mealtimes. Always try to offer healthy snacks, such as pieces of fresh fruit, cheese or unsalted rice cakes, and well-diluted juice or water. Allow a two-hour gap between meals so that your child's appetite is not affected. If he is not hungry at mealtimes, he is more likely to be fussy about his food.

* If possible, you should give a main protein meal at lunchtime when he is more alert and therefore more likely to eat all his food. Then you won't need to worry as much if your child is tired at teatime and becomes fussy about his meal.

* Your child will become more aware of colours and shapes in the second year, and he will enjoy eating food that looks attractive. A selection of different coloured vegetables with his main course is more appealing than having all his food mixed up together.

* Your toddler will probably prefer a variety of foods in small quantities, rather than large amounts of one or two foods. If you give him a selection of foods, it will encourage him to try more of them.

* Be careful not to put too much food on his plate, as this can be off-putting. It is better to serve a smaller amount and give him a second helping if he finishes it all.

* Don't let your child watch TV while he eats – it is important to avoid distractions during mealtimes. Reading or playing games can also distract a child from his food.

* Lots of children of this age like fromage frais, but do be careful with this as many brands contain extremely high levels of sugar. You may find that if your toddler eats a lot of fromage frais, he has less appetite at mealtimes.

* Remember that mealtimes should be happy times. If your toddler begins to associate meals with stress and negative feelings, this can turn a minor problem into a more long-lasting issue.

Case study: Charlotte, aged 14 months
Problem: Refusal of food at lunchtime and teatime
Cause: Imbalance in types of food and snacking

Charlotte had always been a good feeder, and once weaned onto solids she would eat a wide variety of different vegetables and fruit. By seven months of age she was on three good meals a day, happily taking different types of protein at lunchtime, and took easily to different finger foods and chopped food when introduced.

When Charlotte was just over a year old her mother, Lisa, returned to work full time and Charlotte went to nursery five days a week from 8.30am until 5pm. She would have her breakfast at home followed by lunch and tea at the nursery. Within a couple of weeks of Charlotte attending nursery, Lisa noticed that she was becoming more and more fussy about her food, particularly at lunch and teatime. The nursery staff assured Lisa that this behaviour was very normal at around this age and it was a time when many children naturally cut back on the amount of food they ate, as their growth rate slowed down during the second year.

However, over the next few weeks Charlotte's feeding got so bad at lunchtime that she started to scream after a couple of spoonfuls, and she had gone from happily chewing bite-sized pieces of chicken, lamb and fish to refusing all protein whatsoever.

At the nursery teatime of 4pm, Charlotte would eat a little but rarely more than a couple of teaspoons of pasta or some other savoury dish followed by half a bread-stick or rice cake and perhaps a small fromage frais. When her mother picked her up at 5pm she would then try to coax Charlotte to eat because she knew that she had had very little at the nursery. However, the more she tried to get Charlotte to eat, the worse the screaming became. By bedtime Charlotte was normally so exhausted from screaming and fighting that she would fall asleep after drinking only 120–150ml (4–5oz) of her bedtime milk.

By the time she reached 14 months, the only food Charlotte would eat happily was the cereal and toast that she had at breakfast. Lisa, very concerned that Charlotte had refused all forms of animal protein and was eating only tiny amounts of fruit and vegetables for over a month, rang me for advice on how to get her eating happily again.

I asked Lisa to keep a diary of everything that Charlotte ate and drank over the next three days and, very importantly, the times that everything was consumed. I explained that the timing of food and drinks *was probably the cause of Charlotte's refusal to eat meat or fish rather than a sudden dislike of it. The nursery offered tea at 4pm, which, in my opinion, is much too early for a child to have their last meal of the day, particularly if parents do not offer them a snack an hour or so prior to bedtime.*

I was sure that this was the start of Charlotte's problem, and when I received her food diary the amount she was eating confirmed this. Although Lisa did not realise it, Charlotte was eating excessive amounts of food at breakfast. After a drink of 210ml (7oz) of milk, she would eat 2–3 tablespoonfuls of breakfast cereal mixed with milk and fruit, followed by a slice of toast with cheese spread or mashed banana, and would often go on to have a fromage frais. Charlotte's breakfast had steadily become bigger and bigger once her teatime had been brought forward from 5pm to 4pm when she started nursery.

The huge breakfast, along with a drink of juice and a biscuit at 10am, was, I felt, the reason that Charlotte had started to refuse her lunch. As she ate little or no lunch, she was given a drink of milk and a biscuit at 2.30pm. The amount of milk she drank had gradually increased in volume, and it wasn't until the nursery started to measure out the amount being consumed at 2.30pm that they realised it was 210–270ml (7–9oz). This huge amount of milk meant that she would eat only very little when the nursery, and then her mother, tried to feed her between 4pm and 6pm. All this meant that Charlotte was so hungry by the morning that she was taking excessive amounts of food at her first meal of the day. Breakfast filled her up so much that she was not hungry enough for lunch, and a vicious circle soon evolved of her eating and drinking too much of the wrong foods at the wrong time.

I advised Lisa to give Charlotte the same volume of food at breakfast but to make it up from fruit and yoghurt and cut out cereal for three days. Charlotte should not be given a biscuit in the morning, only a drink of juice, and her lunch should be brought forward slightly to 11/11.30am when she would show signs of hunger. Within three days Charlotte was back to eating and enjoying a well-balanced meal of chicken or fish with vegetables and a serving of carbohydrates at lunchtime. This meant that she was no longer hungry at 2.30pm and was happy to take just a drink of well-diluted juice and a piece of fruit. At 4pm she would have tea at the nursery but I advised her mother to request slightly smaller portions for her so that she would then take a second helping of carbohydrates between 5pm and 6pm.

Having something to eat slightly later in the day and taking a larger drink of milk at bedtime meant that

Charlotte did not wake up so hungry in the morning. By the fourth day Lisa reintroduced a serving of breakfast cereal and reduced the fruit. Charlotte also had 150–180ml (5–6oz) of milk.

The problem of suddenly refusing lunch is a fairly common one and is rarely caused by a sudden dislike of protein but by an imbalance in the types of foods, which are often given at the wrong times. I always advise parents to ensure that they enrol their young babies or toddlers in a nursery that is willing to keep a detailed food and fluid diary and that will make minor changes, if necessary, to fit in with an individual child's needs.

The third year

By the time your child is into his third year, if you are not already doing so, you should include him in as many adult meals as possible.

* Aim to offer your child what the rest of the family is eating whenever you can. Children learn by example and he is far more likely to try a food that he sees you eating and enjoying. Lots of praise and encouragement will give him an incentive to eat well. If you are still cooking him separate meals at this stage, you are setting a precedent for him to refuse the food you eat at family meals.

* Encourage your child to sit at the table, using child-sized cutlery and crockery. He should be drinking without help from a normal cup with handles by now. There will inevitably be some accidents and spills, but it is important for him to learn how to pick up a cup and sip from it. If he has real problems with this, he may find it easier to use a straw.

* Encouraging your child to get involved in preparing food when you can is a good idea. He will enjoy helping out in the kitchen, and if you get him involved in choosing and cooking his food, he may be far more willing to try something new.

* At this age, children can become fussy about the look of what they are eating. They like food that they can recognise and may not want foods that are mixed together. Some children get deeply suspicious of things like soups, stews, pies or casseroles where they can't immediately identify all the things they are eating.

* It is worth persevering with new foods. Children will usually be willing to try a little of something, and you can gradually increase the quantities of new foods. If your child is offered food that he hasn't tried before, encourage him to at least taste it rather than refusing it. Explain that he won't have to eat it all up if he doesn't like it, but that he should try it first. If he still refuses, leave it for two or three weeks and then try again.

- If your child is starting nursery at this age, make sure he has a filling breakfast in the morning that includes a good serving of carbohydrate. This will give him the stamina to get through the day and he will be able to concentrate more fully. At the end of his day at nursery, he will be hungry and tired. Try to have food prepared in advance and to be organised with mealtimes so that you don't resort to giving him non-nutritious snacks. This will ruin his appetite for his proper meal, and can lead to fussy eating.

- To encourage your child to eat vegetables, try to offer them in an appealing way. Baby vegetables such as mini carrots, baby sweetcorn, sugar snaps and mange tout are naturally sweet and popular with children. Salads with mini-tomatoes, chopped cucumber and raw carrot often go down well too.

Older children

Children who have started out eating well can sometimes suddenly develop fussy eating habits when they are older.

Remember that this may just be a matter of your child exerting his own independence. If he has eaten well until this stage, fussy eating is generally a phase that he will eventually outgrow.

* Many children start to have their own social lives around the age of three, and will not always be eating with you at home. You may find that your child will eat things at a friend's house or at school that at home he would turn his nose up at – children are often more adventurous in their eating habits when they aren't at home. Tell other parents to offer your child what they would eat, and not to prepare anything special to fit in with any fussy eating habits he may have. This can be a good way of getting children to try foods that they would normally refuse.

* Don't fall into the trap of only feeding your child foods that you think he will eat. Wherever possible, cook what you would like to eat as a family. If you present your child with a wide variety of foods, he is far more likely to be willing to try different things.

- Try to avoid offering your child too many snacks when he gets home from nursery or school. If he is already full-up with snack foods when he sits down to a meal, he is less likely to eat a proper lunch or tea.

- If your child starts to refuse to eat meals, don't allow snacks between meals. Many children would be quite happy to forget about meals and live on snacks, but it is important to establish regular mealtimes if you want to encourage healthy eating and avoid fussiness.

- When your child tries something new to eat, make sure you praise him in just the same way that you would for any other kind of good behaviour.

- Be realistic about how much you can expect your child to eat. If you give him too much food at mealtimes, he will not be able to finish it and will not be praised for this.

- Don't impose your own eating habits on your child. If he likes to eat ketchup with all his vegetables, this isn't the end of the world. It's far better for him to be eating vegetables with ketchup than no vegetables at all.

* Children learn by example, therefore you can't expect your child to eat vegetables if you won't either.

I hope that all of these tips will allow you to feel more confident about your child's eating, and not to worry too much about how much he eats. If you eat well yourself, show your child that you enjoy a variety of foods and encourage him to join you for healthy and nutritious meals at the table, he is far less likely to have any lasting fussiness around food as he grows older.

3
How to Deal with Fussy Eating Problems

It is important to remember that many children will be fussy about food at certain times in their lives, but if the problem becomes more severe and you have a child who is refusing to eat anything other than bread and jam or chicken nuggets at every meal, then you do need to take some remedial action.

Do you have a problem?

Sometimes it is easy to get worried if you don't feel your child eats enough, or if he suddenly starts to reject certain foods. I'd always advise keeping a food diary for a few weeks if you are feeling anxious, as this is the best way to get a true picture of what your child is consuming. You may be surprised to find that although he doesn't eat much at mealtimes, he is eating quite a lot of snacks between meals, or is making up for what he doesn't eat one day by having far more than usual the next day.

You should try to ensure that your child eats something from each of the main food groups (see page 15), but try not to worry if he refuses certain foods. If his diet is broadly balanced, he may still be getting all the essentials he needs. By keeping a food diary you will spot whether there are any gaps in his basic nutritional needs.

If you are really worried, you should check your child is fit and healthy and that there are no underlying medical reasons behind his fussiness about food. Take him to your health visitor or GP to be weighed and measured to make sure that he is growing properly. You may want to ask for a blood test to check his iron levels aren't causing problems. If your food diary has suggested that your child's diet isn't providing the essential nutrients he needs, talk to your GP about using a vitamin or mineral supplement. Remember, however, that this is not an alternative to a healthy diet and that you should consider this a short-term solution.

The basic rules

There are some basic rules you should follow for a fussy eater. If you follow these rules properly and consistently, this may be sufficient to sort out the problem.

* Explain to your child that if he doesn't eat his meals, he will not be offered snacks as an alternative. Always stick to this rule.

- Make sure he is actually hungry at mealtimes, and hasn't filled up on drinks and snacks beforehand.

- Allow him to eat at least half of his food at mealtimes before you offer a drink. Avoid giving him sugary drinks or undiluted fruit juice with his meal.

- Stick to a pattern of regular mealtimes.

- If your child refuses to eat something, don't try to force-feed him and try not to shout or to get upset.

- Keep mealtimes short – around 30 minutes. Don't let them turn into a battle. If your child is continuing to refuse to eat, simply take the plate away.

- If you are feeling anxious about what your child is eating, try not to let him see this. It is all too easy to convey your concerns to your child, which can exacerbate the problem.

Dealing with a fussy eater

In my experience, fussy eating habits can easily become ingrained and it can take time and effort to change your child's attitude to food. I have found that one of the best ways to deal with fussy eating is to take a seemingly relaxed approach, by ignoring the problem and calming the situation before gradually beginning to introduce a wider diet.

Stage one – restoring calm

If things have developed to the stage where mealtimes have booome a source of argument and stress, start by restoring some peace. This in itself can make a difference to the way your child eats, as stress can kill appetite. If your child equates mealtimes with arguments, his stress levels will rise as soon as he sits down at the table. This can lead to the release of hormones which restrict the blood supply to the stomach and can then affect your child's appetite.

* Make sure that the rest of the family are aware of what you are trying to do, although be careful not to say anything about it to your child. It is essential that both parents present a united front on this so that your child doesn't receive conflicting signals. Childminders, nannies or au pairs who may be preparing food for your child should be made aware of what you are doing. If your child's siblings are much older and can understand, you may want to explain to them, but with younger children it will be easier not to say anything at all.

* If the source of stress has been one particular food, for example certain vegetables, then don't serve your child the food he has been refusing. Prepare a normal meal for the rest of the family, but do not give your fussy eater any of the foods that he has issues with.

* At this stage, your child will probably feel he has won the battle and he will start to relax. Don't discuss it with him, but instead act as if nothing has happened.

* You will find that mealtimes become far more relaxing for you, too. Try to let go of all the stress that has built up around mealtimes. You may still be worried about the fact that your child's diet is limited and that he is not eating all that you would like, but take care not to express any of these concerns to your child.

* Continue with this strategy for at least a week or two. By then, mealtimes will have become more enjoyable again and both you and your child should be feeling more relaxed.

Stage two – introducing new foods

It is only once you and your child have become more relaxed that you can start gradually working on expanding your child's diet.

* When you are out shopping with your child, find a food that you know he has never tried but that you enjoy. If your

child has a vegetable problem, you may want to start with something sweet like sweet potato or butternut squash.

* Cook the new food in an appealing way (for example, you could bake slices of sweet potato so that they look like chunky chips), and serve it at the table to everyone else, but don't offer any to your child.

* Talk about the food – about where it comes from and how it grows. You could even search for some fascinating facts related to the food by looking on the Internet. If you can manage to get your child interested, he is more likely to want to taste the food.

* Gradually introduce more new foods, or prepare familiar ones in a new way, and talk about how you've cooked them or where they come from, but do not offer any to your child. At this stage, don't even suggest that he might like to try things that you are cooking.

* If you continue with this, the majority of children will soon cave in and ask to try some of what you are eating. Some may do it sneakily when they think you aren't looking!

* Be patient, it may take time, but the more interesting you make your food sound and the less bothered you appear to be about your child eating it, the more likely he is to want to try whatever you have prepared.

* Remember, your child's bad eating habits may have taken years to establish, and are unlikely to instantly disappear. It can take time and effort as young children can be extremely stubborn.

* Don't forget to praise your child when he eats new foods, just as you would offer praise for other good behaviour. This will help him to feel good about healthy eating. Tell him why they are good for him, for example, 'They'll make you grow big and tall like Daddy' or 'They'll make you one of the fastest runners in nursery.'

How to encourage your child to eat more vegetables

Many parents have difficulty getting their child to eat five portions of fruit and vegetables a day, and some children will refuse to eat any vegetables at all. If your child rejects vegetables, try to encourage him to eat more fruit to make up for this, but with a little imagination, you may be able to make vegetables more appealing.

* Some children don't like cooked vegetables, but prefer to eat them raw and will eat grated carrot or chopped tomatoes.

* Chop up some crunchy vegetables such as carrot, cucumber or peppers into sticks and serve with a dip such as hummus or salsa.

* Try placing a plate of chopped vegetables and a dip on the table when your child gets home from school or nursery. Make sure they are somewhere that your child will see them, but don't make an issue about it. It may help if you try this when your child has a friend round who you know

eats well, as your child will be more likely to eat if he sees his friend enjoying the vegetables.

* Add sliced or puréed vegetables to pasta sauces, casseroles or stews.

* Stir-fry vegetables with some meat, fish or chicken for a Chinese-style meal.

* Mash cooked carrot, peas, sweetcorn or swede with potatoes and serve as a spread on rice cakes or as a filler in pitta bread.

* Grilled cheese and tomato on a slice of bread or pitta makes a good snack.

* Serve sliced vegetables with sandwiches.

* If your toddler refuses to eat vegetables, try puréeing vegetable soup very smoothly and adding some cool, boiled water or milk. Give it as a drink from a cup.

* Try introducing some recipes that use a combination of fruit and vegetables such as Chicken-peach Casserole (see page 105) and Fruity Lamb Tagine (see page 102).

* Look for recipes that use hidden vegetables.

Case study: Alfie, aged 4
Problem: Refusal of vegetables

Although Alfie ate well as a baby, he was never very keen on vegetables. During the first stage of weaning, Alfie would fuss and fret when given vegetable purées but would happily gobble up any type of fruit purée. By the time he reached one year of age he would only ever eat carrots, peas or sweetcorn, and occasionally small amounts of sweet potato.

Just before his second birthday, Alfie began to get more and more picky about his food; he started to refuse meals that he had eaten happily before, and he cut out sweet potato and sweetcorn altogether. The only vegetables he would eat now were carrots and peas – and even then he would only eat them if there were smothered with tomato ketchup.

Alfie and his mother, Chrissie, led a hectic social life and attended lots of play dates during his second year, which often included lunch or tea. Many of Chrissie's friends were experiencing similar problems of picky eating, and rather than face a massive protest at mealtime from their children, a habit of lunch or tea at McDonald's or Burger King was quickly established.

By the time Alfie reached his third birthday his meals consisted mainly of chicken nuggets or fish fingers served with processed potato shapes and baked beans, carrots or peas with lots of ketchup, or a burger and fries with ketchup on the days they ate out.

His normal breakfast cereal of Weetabix or Shreddies and fruit had also become replaced with cereals, such as Frosties and Coco Pops, which he had discovered during a weekend away with friends.

Although deep down Chrissie was becoming increasingly worried about the limited variety and lack of healthy foods that Alfie was now eating, friends assured her that the majority of children went through this phase and that once Alfie was attending nursery for the full day and eventually going to school, his interest in a large variety of foods would improve.

Chrissie allowed things to continue but, as Alfie neared his fourth birthday, she grew more worried. She had noticed a huge difference in his behaviour over the previous few months. He had always been a very gentle, easy-going little boy, but now she noticed that he was becoming more and more irritable and much more prone to sudden outbursts of temper especially at mealtimes. Chrissie realised that she was going to have to do something about Alfie's diet. She was convinced that he was not getting all the nutrients he needed from the limited types of foods that he was eating and she was sure that his increasingly bad behaviour was also related to his diet.

That afternoon at a play date she discussed her fears with the other mothers, and one suggested that she contact me.

When Chrissie and I spoke, it was obvious that she was distressed and feeling very guilty that she might have done Alfie some damage by allowing him to eat such a restricted diet for so long. I reassured her that while his diet was very limited, I was sure that over a period of several days his nutritional requirements were not as deficient as she thought they were. I told her to continue to feed Alfie as usual but to keep a diary of absolutely everything he ate and drank over the next four days. It was also important to give exact details of the amounts and the times of everything consumed.

I usually find with young children who eat a very limited diet, and particularly those who refuse to eat vegetables, that they are eating either excessive carbohydrates or protein, which can often contribute to the problem of refusal to eat vegetables and can limit their interest in a wider variety of foods. When Chrissie sent me the food diary, three things immediately stood out. First, Alfie was eating a very generous amount of protein at both lunch and tea. Although his diet was certainly very limited, usually fish fingers or chicken nuggets, Alfie had, over a four-day period, consumed the equivalent of 10 portions of protein per day, much more than the daily requirement. Second, he was generally consuming excessive amounts of carbohydrate, which were filling him up. Third, he was eating too few vegetables.

Although an unbalanced diet is not the only cause of poor eating habits or a refusal of vegetables, overloading a child with too much of a particular food group can contribute to the problem. I sent Chrissie a list of foods and information about what constitutes a portion. I advised her that she should not attempt to change Alfie's diet just yet, but to limit the amount of proteins and carbohydrates to the recommended daily amounts (see pages 15–17). At the same time, she was to offer him a choice of vegetables at each meal. I suggested that she and Alfie should go to the shops together and that he should help choose what vegetables he would like for the following two days. It was also important that Chrissie spent time discussing with Alfie why vegetables are important, for example, that carrots will help him to have good eyesight for watching his favourite video, so it is important that he eats a small amount of carrots every week; and broccoli, peppers and cauliflower will help him to grow big and tall like Daddy.

I also advised Chrissie to bring colours and shapes into meal preparation, for example, mixing some tiny green peas with some orange slices of carrot.

During the first week of reintroducing vegetables into Alfie's diet, I advised Chrissie not to be tempted to overload his plate with the same types, even if he showed signs of wanting to eat more. It was better to start off with only two slices of carrot and one broccoli floret and gradually build it up over a period of a couple of weeks than to overload his plate and risk him rejecting it. The majority of children can be persuaded to eat two slices of carrot or one teaspoon of sweetcorn. Every few days it can be increased by such a tiny amount that they rarely notice, and after a couple of weeks they will be happily eating proper portions.

I also explained that it was very important for Chrissie to sit down and eat with Alfie whenever possible. I believe that many eating problems evolve because children reach a stage where they feel very threatened when left sitting alone to eat a plate of food. They cannot understand why they should be expected to eat all the different foods on their plate when Mummy and Daddy are rushing about and only having to eat a sandwich.

Chrissie made a point of always eating breakfast and, whenever possible, lunch with Alfie, and within a couple of weeks he had started to eat small amounts of vegetables with his lunch and tea. I felt it was now time to resolve the problem of him wanting to eat only chicken nuggets and fish fingers. I advised her to buy a cookery book with recipes written especially for children. They should look at the book together and choose a special recipe to cook for Daddy at the weekend. Alfie decided he liked the look of mini pizza, so on Saturday morning

Chrissie helped him to prepare and cook the pizza, reading the recipe out step by step. A quick visit to the kitchen from Daddy, who hinted that he would love some green and red peppers on the top, also went down well and encouraged Alfie to have a small taste of something new.

I advised Chrissie to continue encouraging Alfie to help shop and prepare a new meal twice a week, once for Daddy and once for his special friends. I also suggested that Chrissie cut out nice pictures of different dishes from magazines and paste them in a scrapbook. It was called 'Alfie's Special Recipe Book'. Alongside the pictures Chrissie would write simple instructions, which she would read to Alfie as they prepared the meals together. Of course she sometimes had to adapt certain recipes, and sometimes they were given new names. Naming the recipes after characters from your children's favourite video or story-book or a favourite friend or relation will also help to keep their enthusiasm.

It took a further two months for Chrissie to expand on Alfie's range of foods, but she felt all the hard work and effort were worth it as he now eats a healthy diet.

While it is important that a child is never forced to eat foods that he genuinely dislikes, I believe that with the huge variety of foods available, particularly vegetables and salads, it is not acceptable that a child dislikes every single one. Refusal of vegetables is a very common problem among young children and can be avoided if parents give their children a choice and refuse to substitute them repeatedly with the same favoured foods.

How to encourage your child to eat more fruit

✿ Make fruit smoothies with a mixture of fresh fruit.

✿ Serve fruit in slices with a dip such as flavoured yoghurt, or occasionally with ice cream as a special treat.

✿ Slice bananas and add to your child's favourite breakfast cereal.

✿ Chop up some fruit into bite-sized pieces for a snack, or in a lunchbox, rather than including whole fruit.

✿ Serve some canned fruit (in natural juice, not syrup) with yoghurt.

✿ Chop some fruit and leave it on a plate in the fridge at your child's eye-level. This will encourage him to eat a piece if he opens the fridge looking for a snack.

✿ Make a crumble or pie using lots of fruit.

✿ Look for recipes that use hidden fruit.

Healthy snacking

Eating too many snacks can often lead to problems at meal-times. It is difficult for young children to eat large quantities at meals and they are so active that they often need the added fuel of snacks between meals. However, if they have too many snacks, or the wrong type of snacks, this can end up affecting their overall diet.

* Children should not be eating crisps, chocolate or sweets on a regular basis as they are high in fat, sugar and salt. If your child is hungry when you are out, it is sometimes difficult to find healthy snacks and it is easy to resort to junk food, but this is not appropriate for growing children, especially if it is done on a regular basis.

* If your child doesn't eat a meal, and you offer snacks later in the day as an alternative, he may not eat his next meal. This can quickly become a problem, with a child refusing meals and living on snacks instead. This will be a serious problem if your child is eating high fat, sugary or salty snack foods.

- Fruit is always a good snack choice. You may want to chop up fruit for small children, but taking a banana or some grapes with you when you go out means that you always have a healthy snack on hand.

- Breadsticks or rice cakes are good snacks for a child. Don't give too much close to mealtimes as they are filling and may mean that your child won't eat well.

- Add your own flavourings, such as chopped-up fruit, to natural yoghurt for an excellent snack food. Shop-bought flavoured yoghurts can be high in sugar.

- Cubes or cut-up strips of cheese are often popular with children, and are a good source of calcium. Too much cheese can quickly fill a child up though, so don't give too much close to mealtimes.

- Chopped vegetables with dips are a great snack food. Carrot or celery sticks are often popular with children who refuse to eat cooked vegetables.

If you have a fussy eater in the family, do remember that you will need to be patient. This is not always something that you can resolve instantly, but if you are willing to persevere, you will find that your child gradually becomes more willing to try new foods.

4
Encouraging an Interest in Food

Children who are encouraged to get involved when their parents are food shopping, and who lend a hand with preparing meals, do tend to develop a healthy interest in food. Fussy eating habits are less common among children who regularly engage in these activities, and involving a fussy eater in food shopping and cooking can often help solve the problem.

Talk to your child about the meals he likes best and what goes into them, take him with you to the shops and let him 'help' in the kitchen whenever you can do this safely and easily (see page 88). It will enable him to feel more involved in what he is eating and he will be happier to try new foods if he has helped to choose or cook them himself.

Older pre-school children may enjoy drawing up menu plans for the family, or creating recipe books by cutting out pictures from magazines. They will also enjoy simple baking (see page 96), and an afternoon spent at home in the kitchen making healthy muffins, biscuits or bread can be great fun for all the family.

Shopping with children

Food shopping with young children doesn't have to be a chore. Your child will enjoy shopping if you take a little more time over it, and allow him to be involved. He will enjoy putting items into your basket or trolley, and helping to choose what you buy.

* Try to avoid shopping trips when your child is tired or hungry as it won't be an enjoyable experience.

* Make sure you have a supply of nutritious snacks with you for a toddler. Otherwise you may end up buying him something unhealthy because you are in a hurry to satisfy his hunger.

* Discuss what you need with your child as you go round the shop. If you can, let him make some choices himself as he will really enjoy this. You could say that you want to try a new type of fruit or vegetable, and let him pick which you will buy. Children are far more likely to try something new if they have helped to choose it.

* Explain what things are as you shop, which countries they come from and what they are used for. It will help your child develop an understanding of what goes into his meals.

* Try to use local greengrocers, butchers or fishmongers now and again rather than only shopping in the supermarket. It may take a little more time, but it is often a far more interesting experience for your child.

* Visiting a local market can be great fun for a child, and cheaper for you, too.

* If your child is going to bake or cook something with you, it is a good idea to get him involved right from the start of the process by taking him shopping with you to purchase the ingredients.

Helping with food preparation

Cooking is often a task that parents perform alone, without thinking to involve their children. Obviously, getting your child to help when you are in a rush to get a meal ready is not a good idea, so wait until you have a little more time to go at your child's pace. He will enjoy simple tasks, such as passing you ingredients, and is more likely to eat a meal that he has played a role in preparing.

Even quite young children may be able to help by:

* Getting fruit from the bowl or vegetables from the vegetable rack.
* Washing fruit and vegetables.
* Taking tins out of the cupboard.
* Arranging chopped vegetables on a plate.
* Helping with spooning, pouring and measuring ingredients.
* Tearing up lettuce or cabbage leaves, or breaking up broccoli florets.

Young children can practise chopping on soft fruit such as bananas or kiwi fruit using a table knife and older ones could try soft vegetables such as mushrooms or courgettes. Explain that knives can be dangerous – show your child how to use the knife properly and safely and make sure you supervise at all times.

While you are cooking

Safety in the kitchen is paramount, and you do have to be very careful with young children when they are near a hot oven, steaming kettle or sharp knives. However, as long as you have time to do things carefully, children can really benefit from being involved in cooking a family meal.

* Explain to your child what you are doing as you go along, so that he can see the ingredients that go into the food he enjoys.

* Get your child to start by washing his hands thoroughly, and explain the importance of this beforehand.

* An apron will help protect your child's clothes as cooking is often a messy business with young children. Make sure sleeves are rolled up and long hair is tied back.

* If possible, let him help by passing you ingredients as you cook. Count out the different fruit or vegetables together and discuss the colours and shapes.

* Show him how you weigh things on scales, and explain the measures. This is a useful lesson for your child.

* He may enjoy helping to whisk or mix, but you should allow a little extra time for this!

* If there is a simple task he could do, encourage him to join in. Older children could grease a cake tin, butter bread or help lay the table.

* It is important to be aware of safety in the kitchen at all times. Make sure your child keeps away from the oven or hob, never leave the handles of pans turned outwards when they are on the stove and keep your child away from any sharp or potentially dangerous kitchen implements. Never leave a child unattended in the kitchen.

A simple family recipe

This recipe is popular with most children and is easy to prepare. You can put pretty much anything on top of a pizza, and children enjoy choosing their own toppings and creating their own mini-pizzas.

Pizza

Makes 4 small pizzas

For the base

750g (1½lb) strong bread flour
7g (0.3oz) sachet fast-action yeast
½ teaspoon salt
425ml (14½oz) warm water
1 tablespoon clear honey
2 tablespoons olive oil

* Put the flour, yeast and salt into a large mixing bowl.
* Put the warm water into a jug and stir in the honey and oil.

✿ Add the liquid to the flour and mix it until you have a soft dough. You may need to add a little extra water if it is too dry.

✿ Put the dough on to a floured board, and knead it for five to 10 minutes. Children will love doing this, and they can't really spoil it at this stage, so encourage them to have a go.

✿ Once it feels smooth and springy, you can leave the dough to rise in a warm place until it has doubled in size. You can make the sauce while the dough is rising.

For the sauce

1 tablespoon olive oil
1 large or 2 small onions, finely chopped
2 garlic cloves, finely chopped
400g (14oz) can chopped tomatoes
350g (12oz) jar passata
1 teaspoon dried mixed herbs
½ teaspoon sugar

- Heat the oil in a heavy-based pan, and add the onions. Cook over a medium heat until they are soft.

- Add the garlic, and cook for another minute before putting in the remaining ingredients.

- Stir well and bring to the boil, then leave to simmer, uncovered, on a gentle heat for 10–15 minutes.

- Once the sauce is thickened, it is ready.

You can add other vegetables to this sauce – a very finely chopped or grated carrot, a sliced courgette or pepper, even grated beetroot – and then blend the sauce before using it on the pizza. This can be a good way of ensuring your child eats more vegetables!

To make the pizzas

- Pre-heat the oven to 200°C/180°C fan-assisted oven/Gas Mark 6.

- Divide the dough into four.

* Roll out each piece to make a flat pizza base. Put them on a greased baking tray and bake them for five minutes.

* Remove them from the oven and cover with a layer of sauce, followed by whatever toppings your child has chosen.

* Return to the oven and bake for another 10 minutes.

Some pizza topping suggestions

Children will really enjoy choosing their own pizza toppings, and can come up with some slightly unusual combinations, but as long as they are happy to eat whatever they've chosen, that isn't a problem. Here are some suggestions:

* Mozzarella cheese
* Ham
* Tuna
* Sliced green, red or yellow peppers
* Sliced mushrooms

* Thinly sliced courgette or carrot

* Florets of blanched broccoli

* Sweetcorn

* Sliced tomatoes or halved cherry tomatoes

Baking together

Children love baking, and spending an hour or so together making healthy cup cakes, biscuits or savoury muffins can be a really rewarding activity for you both.

* Make sure you are prepared – have all the ingredients you need to hand.

* Younger children will enjoy spooning ingredients into the mixing bowl and stirring, while older ones will be able to help measure out the ingredients too.

* Biscuits are fun for children, especially if you have a selection of cookie cutters. You may need to roll out the dough,

but they will enjoy cutting out the biscuits. Don't be too fussy about odd shapes – your children won't mind.

✿ Remember that your child will never learn to do things if you don't let him try. There will inevitably be flour on the floor and cake mix on the table the first time he makes cakes, but this is all part of the learning process. Let him do as much as he can himself as this will give him a far greater sense of satisfaction.

Washing up

It may be a chore to you, but young children love nothing more than a bowl of bubbly water.

✿ Make sure the water is warm and not hot.

✿ If your child can't reach the sink safely on a stable chair, you may want to give him a bowl of water at the table for his 'washing up', but you will have spillages so make sure the surface is protected.

- Use a mild washing-up liquid as some can dry out the skin and may not be ideal for a young child.

- Dress your child in a waterproof apron and get him to roll up his sleeves before he starts.

- Give him a brush or sponge, and show him how to use it.

- Let him wash a few 'safe' items – plastic bowls, spatulas or wooden spoons.

- He may then want to dry the things he's washed with a tea towel.

Popular recipes

Many parents have told me that the following recipes are popular with their toddlers. Try them with your child, and encourage him to help with the preparation. For more recipes, see *The Contented Little Baby Book of Weaning*, *The Gina Ford Baby and Toddler Cook Book* and *Feeding Made Easy*.

Baby Bolognese

Makes 4–6 servings

150g (5oz) extra-lean minced beef steak
1 small onion, peeled and finely chopped
75g (3oz) button mushrooms, wiped and sliced
200g (7oz) carrots, peeled and diced
150g (5oz) courgettes, diced
a few stems of fresh marjoram or large pinch of
  dried marjoram
oil for frying
600ml (1 pint) home-made chicken stock or boiling
  filtered water
75g (3oz) soup pasta
2 tablespoons tomato purée (optional)

✿ Dry-fry the meat and onion together in a saucepan until browned. Stir-fry the other vegetables with a little oil. Remove from the heat and add the herbs and stock or water. Return to the heat, cover and bring to the boil, then lower the heat and simmer for 30 minutes, stirring occasionally, until beef and vegetables are tender.

* Meanwhile, cook pasta in a saucepan of boiling water for 6–7 minutes (or according to packet instructions) or until tender. Drain well.

* Mix the beef and pasta together and stir in the tomato purée, if using.

Tips

* As beef has a strong taste, use slightly less than other meats until your toddler is happy with this new flavour.

Chicken and Parmesan Fingers

Makes 1–2 servings

1 large boneless, skinless chicken breast
90ml (3oz) full-fat milk, mixed with 1 dessertspoon runny
  honey
1 tablespoon olive oil
1 egg, beaten
1 tablespoon freshly grated Parmesan cheese, mixed
  with 2 tablespoons breadcrumbs

* Cut the chicken into strips and marinade in the milk and honey mixture for 1 hour.

* Pour the oil into a frying pan and bring to sizzling point. Meanwhile, dip the chicken strips into the beaten egg and then into the cheese and breadcrumb mixture, before adding to the pan.

* Cook for 5 minutes on each side or until the chicken is cooked through and golden and crispy.

Tip

✿ Serve with Vegetable Dippers or any of the recipes in the vegetables chapter from *The Gina Ford Baby and Toddler Cook Book*.

Fruity Lamb Tagine

To freeze this dish, divide it into separate portions for all the family, place in airtight containers and freeze for up to a month.

Makes 6–8 servings

25g (1oz) unsalted butter
1 medium onion, peeled and finely chopped
450g (1lb) lean lamb, diced
1 tbsp plain flour
2 medium carrots, peeled and sliced
400g (14oz) can of chopped tomatoes with herbs

200g (7oz) dried apricots, chopped
50g (2oz) sultanas
150ml (5oz) vegetable stock

* In a large, lidded saucepan, melt the butter, add the onion and cook for 2–3 minutes. Coat the lamb in the flour, add to the onion and cook for a further 3–4 minutes, stirring continuously, until the meat is browned all over.

* Add the carrots, tomatoes, dried fruit and stock and bring to the boil, then turn the heat down and cover with the lid. Simmer very gently for about 1 hour or until the lamb is tender.

* Serve with rice or couscous.

Quick Salmon Fishcakes

Makes 6 fishcakes

4 medium potatoes, peeled
50g (2oz) unsalted butter
200g (7oz) tin of red salmon
1 tsp freshly squeezed lemon juice
1 egg yolk, beaten
1 egg white, beaten
75g (3oz) breadcrumbs
1 tablespoon olive oil

- Boil the potatoes until tender, then mash well, adding a third of the butter, and set aside to cool.

- Add the salmon, lemon juice and egg yolk to the potatoes and mix well. Form into six patties, then coat with beaten egg white, followed by the breadcrumbs.

- Fry gently in the remaining butter and the oil for 3–4 minutes per side or until crispy.

Chicken-peach Casserole

Makes 6–8 servings

> 2 skinless, boneless chicken breast fillets, cubed
> 1 tablespoon unsalted butter
> 1 tablespoon olive oil
> 1 small onion, peeled and chopped
> 2 small carrots, peeled and diced
> 1 small green pepper, deseeded and chopped
> 8 cherry tomatoes, halved
> 150ml (¼ pint) home-made chicken or vegetable stock, or
>   filtered water
> 200g (7oz) can sliced peaches in natural juice

* Wash the chicken breasts under cold running water and dry with kitchen towel.

* Heat the butter and oil in a large frying pan, add the chicken and fry for 3–4 minutes or until brown. Transfer the chicken pieces to a casserole dish.

* Sweat the onion, carrots and green pepper in the remainder of the oil and butter for approximately 7–8 minutes, then add the tomato halves and the stock, and bring to the boil. Pour the peaches and juice or extra stock or water over the chicken pieces. Cover the casserole and cook for 30 minutes.

* Serve with rice or pasta.

Tips

* Rather than canned fruit, use 125g (4oz) ready-to-eat peaches, cut into strips and add an extra 150ml (¼ pint) stock or water.

* Serve with easy-cook brown rice or soup pasta for extra texture.

Case study: Liam, aged 2 years and 10 months
Problem: Sibling rivalry, erratic behaviour and excessive night-time waking
Cause: Using commercially made meals

Serena contacted me a couple of months after the birth of her twin girls. Both babies were doing well on the Contented Little Baby routines, sleeping until 4am from their last feed at 10.30pm. However, since the birth of the twins, their older brother, Liam, had started to wake up two or three times a night, often staying awake for an hour or so at a time. Serena was at breaking point, trying to survive on two to three hours of broken sleep a night and to cope with two babies and a very irritable toddler during the day. Since the birth of the babies, Liam had gone from being an extremely placid, loving little boy to one who would get angry and aggressive, frequently having outbursts of uncontrollable behaviour.

Her health visitor reassured Serena that Liam was probably feeling very insecure and jealous, suddenly finding that he had to share Mummy with not just one baby but two. She arranged for Serena to get some help with the twins twice a week from a government programme in her area called Sure Start so that she could give Liam some undivided attention. Things did improve slightly, but Liam still continued to wake up in the night and would settle back to sleep only when given a drink of fruit juice. He also continued to have uncontrollable outbursts once or twice a day. During one of these outbursts Liam scratched one baby's face so badly that she had to be taken to hospital to have the wound treated. It was at this point that Serena called me to see if I could offer any advice on how to deal with Liam's jealousy and rages.

Regardless of the type of problem a parent is experiencing and wants my help with, I always ask them to send me a feeding and sleeping diary. In my experience, a huge number of the varied problems that parents contact me about tend to be linked in some way to diet. Serena assured me that Liam had always eaten well and was given a wide variety of different foods. The only change in his diet was that she was unable to cook him as many fresh meals as she used to, and, more often than not, he would be given what she and her husband were having for lunch or dinner. In between meals he was only ever given fresh fruit and well-diluted juice.

At first glance it appeared that Liam was eating healthy food – plenty of bread, pasta and rice, along with a wide variety of different vegetables. Every day he would have chicken, fish or lamb at his main meal, *and in the evening he would be given either a pasta dish or thick soup with sandwiches.*

Serena assured me that this was the pattern of eating he had followed since reaching his first birthday. The only difference was that, following the birth of the twins, she did not have time to prepare as much of the food herself, but she always ensured that she did buy the best-quality commercially prepared food. She also admitted that she was allowing Liam to drink fruit squash, something that he had never had in the past.

I asked her to send me a list of the commercially prepared meals and food that she was using. I purchased everything that Serena mentioned on her list and spent a morning analysing the labels and the ingredients. Although experts are divided about the effect commercially prepared food can have on young children, I am convinced that excessive amounts of such foods can adversely affect their behaviour.

When I compared the commercial version with a home-made version of the same dish, I found additional starch fillers and sugars. While an occasional meal containing these things would not affect the behaviour of the majority of children, I believe that, given on a daily basis, they possibly could. This would apply particularly to a child such as Liam, who had always been given meals that consisted of pure, fresh food without fillers, additives and suchlike. Starch fillers, maltodextrin and sugars are of no nutritional benefit to young children, and the main reason they are used is to boost the calorie content of the meal. This means that a child who is fed exclusively on these types of meals would probably not be receiving a properly balanced diet. A well-balanced diet consisting of *a variety of foods is essential for the healthy growth of both mind and body.*

The food diary also showed that Liam was drinking several large cups of fruit squash and eating so-called healthy cereal and milk bars each day. There are many types of fruit drink on the market, which claim to be tooth-friendly and contain no added sugar or artificial colour, and many cereal bars make claims to have similar health benefits.

Once Serena had a clearer understanding of what was in the types of food that Liam was eating, I explained to her how the excessive amounts of refined carbohydrate and sugar in his diet were probably affecting his blood sugar balance, causing him to have erratic mood swings and excessive night-time waking.

I explained to Serena that the problem could not be solved overnight as we would gradually have to wean

Liam off all the highly refined food he was having back onto a well-balanced diet of complex carbohydrates, proteins and fats. His sugary snacks and fruit drinks needed to be replaced with healthier alternatives, such as well-diluted fruit juice and fresh fruit, whole grain rice cakes with a spread or homemade muffins or flapjacks.

The first thing I advised Serena to do was to replace all commercial snacks and drinks with healthier alternatives. Although Liam did have several tantrums about this, they were no worse than his behaviour before we started the change in his diet. By the end of the first week he was having only the fruit drink when he woke in the night, and all his daytime drinks were either water or very well-diluted juice. He was also happily eating healthier snacks and joining in the cooking of home-made treats such as muffins.

During the second week Serena started to replace the commercial meals with similar home-made recipes. Again Liam made a fuss at mealtimes, and on two occasions would not eat lunch. Serena was strong and did not give in to his demands, and by the end of the week he was having home-made meals at both lunch and tea. We then started to introduce healthier cereal options at breakfast, which proved difficult because Liam refused them. Serena did offer him alternatives of toast and spread, or fruit and yoghurt, but for five days Liam refused breakfast. Serena found this very difficult, as she was sure that not having breakfast was nutritionally damaging. I reassured her that she must not feel guilty as she was not starving Liam or refusing him food – she was giving him a choice of healthy options, and by giving in to his demands she could end up with him backtracking to a diet of unhealthy food, which in the long term would do him much more damage. It was a real battle of wills, but by the end of the week Liam was happy to eat one of the healthy breakfast cereals that he was offered.

He was now eating a very healthy diet, but was still prone to emotional outbursts, and although his number of wakings in the night reduced to only one a week, Serena was disappointed that she was still having problems. I explained to her that while Liam's diet was the main cause of his bad behaviour and night-time waking, these problems were also caused by habit, and it could take a long time for things to improve totally.

I suggested that she introduced a star chart to encourage Liam to sleep through the night without having the fruit drink, and for occasions when he behaved particularly well or performed tasks without a fuss.

Although it took a further three weeks to crack the nights, Liam did start to sleep right through the night and his behaviour saw a rapid improvement, with only the occasional temper tantrum (which is normal). He continues to be a very happy little boy who eats a really healthy diet. Serena and I went on to compile a healthy menu plan so that she could do a batch cook once a fortnight and combine healthy frozen meals with quick, fresh alternatives such as risotto, pasta and stir-fries.

Family mealtimes

If your child sees that food is something the rest of the family enjoys, and he is able to join in with this himself, he is far less likely to become fussy about what he eats. Sitting down for a meal together as a family is an important part of this. Children learn by example, and if your child sees other family members eating healthy, nutritious meals rather than living on unhealthy snack foods, he will follow this pattern.

You don't have to spend time making elaborate family meals – plain, simple cooking is what many children enjoy. For some working parents, it isn't possible to have meals with their children during the week, but if you eat together as a family whenever you can, you will find that this not only encourages healthy eating habits but also ensures that you have some family time together which will prove invaluable as your children get older.

5
Frequently Asked Questions

Q My son is 13 months old and I am giving him one breast-feed and two stage-one formula feeds (of 210ml/7oz each) as well as dairy foods each day. I was planning to keep him on formula stage one until 18 months and then switch to cow's milk. Should I be doing it sooner or should I be switching to a next stage formula?

A There's no harm in giving your son formula until he is 18 months old, but if he is eating well, there's also no harm in switching to cow's milk now that he is over the age of one. It will also save you money. If you choose formula, I suggest you switch to the follow-on type as it is higher in iron – which can be lacking if your son does not have a great appetite – and in a number of other nutrients.

It's difficult to know how much breast milk your son is drinking. However, keep in mind that the guideline for daily milk/formula intake at this age is a minimum of 350ml (12oz) and a maximum of 500ml (17oz), including milk used in cereal, yoghurt, cheese and other dairy foods. As your son has 420ml (14oz) formula plus a breast-feed each day in addition to other dairy foods, I suspect he may be over the suggested amount. This is not uncommon, but the problem is that too much milk/formula can reduce your son's intake of the solid foods that provide other nutrients. Now your son is over the age of one it is a good time to aim for a more adult eating pattern – this will probably decrease your son's demand for milk.

I'd suggest offering a nutritious snack (see page 81) mid-afternoon followed by a smaller drink. As it is also about four hours between breakfast and lunch, you could consider a small snack mid-morning. You might also reduce the amount of formula offered and you'll probably find his appetite for solid foods will naturally increase. Another option is to offer drinks of water. Making the change from a bottle to a cup, if you have not done so already, often leads to a reduction in formula/milk intake.

Q **My toddler has become very fussy about drinking his milk, and I have been advised to increase the amount of cheese and yoghurt I give him. As I do not know what a small pot of yoghurt or piece of cheese is equal to in milk amounts, I am unsure how much extra to give him.**

A While it's not difficult to estimate food portions or suitable amounts for adults, it is trickier when you're looking at toddler-sized portions. As a rule of thumb, 210ml of milk (a medium-sized cup or about 7oz) is equivalent to 125g of yoghurt (4½oz, or the size of most small potatoes) or about 30g of cheese (1oz, or a piece about the size of a matchbox). Thus, for smaller eaters, 100ml of milk (about 3½oz) will be equal to a half-tub of yoghurt (or the size of some smaller tubs marketed for young children), or to 14g (½oz) of cheese. In terms of tablespoons of yoghurt, two tablespoons of yoghurt will be approximately equal to three tablespoons of milk (50ml or 2oz), or to about 7g of cheese (0.3oz).

Q **My daughter is almost three years old. What should I give her to drink apart from milk? She has squash (sugar-free) but I am wondering if this is the cause of her very loose poos?**

A I doubt that the sugar-free squash is giving your daughter loose poos. There is a type of sweetener (not an artificial sweetener but a chemical 'relative' of sugar) that can cause diarrhoea if we eat a lot of it. However, it is not used in drinks.

In terms of young children's drinks, apart from milk and water there are three main choices: sugary drinks such as regular squash or fizzy drinks, artificially sweetened drinks such as sugar-free squash, or pure juices and smoothies. All three taste sweet, and one of my concerns is that children who become accustomed to sweet drinks will, as they drink less milk, grow up to only want sweet drinks. A recent report in the *Journal of the American Dietetic Association* reveals that drinks (other than alcohol) supply half of the added sugar and more than a fifth of the calories consumed by US citizens. That's not how I would like to see children grow up – I hope they'll eat nutritious food instead.

As a precautionary measure, it is recommended that children do not consume large amounts of foods containing artificial sweeteners. However, UK studies have, in the past, found that toddlers aged one and a half to four and a half who were consuming the highest amount of artificially sweetened squashes could be exceeding recommended limits for certain artificial sweeteners. While they found that it was unlikely children would come to any harm, advice was issued that these drinks should be diluted more for children than they are for adults. Also, children aged one to four should not have more than three cups a day of drinks containing the artificial sweetener cyclamate (E952). The bottom line: while artificial sweeteners may be safe in limited amounts, most parents are keen that their children consume fewer additives rather than more.

Regular squash and fizzy drinks contain added sugar, and research shows that children and young people in the UK consume too much sugar. Studies have found that children who have consumed a lot of sugary drinks are more likely to be overweight, and health experts are also concerned about links between drinks containing added sugar and the development of diabetes. While there's nothing wrong with children having a little sugar, putting it in the form of a drink makes it easy for children to consume large amounts at once. As well as the health problems already mentioned, regularly drinking sugary drinks may reduce children's appetite for more nutritious foods, make them reluctant to eat non-sweet food and also contribute to tooth decay.

Pure juice and smoothies seem like a much healthier option – they do contain a wealth of vitamins and, in limited amounts, they can be a great asset when children are reluctant to eat fruit. However it's important to realise that, in large amounts, they are equivalent to drinking a sweet, sugary drink. If children are drinking juice or smoothies as a main drink, their bodies will not be able to use all the vitamins in them, but will still absorb all the fruit sugar. And the sugar from juice is also more likely to damage teeth than that in the whole fruit.

Apart from water and milk (in recommended amounts) I believe the best other option is diluting pure juice or smoothie with water. However I suggest gradually reducing the amount of juice and aiming to get as close to pure water as possible*. This will take time and maybe endurance of some protests from your child, but it's her health you're promoting in the long run. Sweet drinks then become a treat for when you're out, such as a juice or smoothie at a cafe, or special occasions at home – a health plan for your wallet as well as your child!

An exception is children who do not eat their recommended five portions of fruit and vegetables each day. They could include a total of one small glass (100ml/3½oz) of pure fruit juice or smoothie diluted with water each day, preferably at mealtimes to reduce damage to their teeth.

Q **My daughter is aged just over two and has always been good with food. But this morning she refused Weetabix. She then asked to have a spoon of my corn-flakes and I said 'no' as it was Mum's breakfast. Should I be offering her a choice now?**

A There's nothing like the terrible twos to make a child want to assert her independence. It's also natural that she will want to copy her mum (who is setting a great example by eating with her toddler), and, having learned about the wide and wonderful world of different foods on offer, to want to enjoy a range of flavours. Unfortunately your more predictable world of knowing what food she will eat for breakfast has now gone out the window, which means breakfast will take that much longer! It also means you'll need to have several suitable options on offer. In addition, I'd recommend vetting your own breakfast choices – as you have seen this morning, Mummy's food will often be the most appealing.

When looking at breakfast cereal, many mums automatically check sugar content. It can be as high as 38g (1¼oz) of sugar per 100g (3½oz) of cereal, meaning over a third of the actual cereal is pure sugar, so this is something to keep an eye on. I'd also suggest monitoring the salt content. Keeping in mind that the daily salt limit for two-year-olds is 2g a day (0.8g sodium), it's worrying that the 30g (1oz) cereal serving that many toddlers would scoff quite easily can contain up to a quarter of a toddler's daily maximum salt intake (0.2g sodium or 0.5g salt). However there are many healthier breakfast cereals on supermarket shelves; it's just a matter of checking the labels. One last thing to watch for is cereals containing whole nuts or large chunks of them, which pose choking and allergy risks.

Some child- and adult-friendly breakfast options other than packaged cereals include:

* Poached egg on toast.

* Porridge – mix in some small raisins and chopped dried apricots for fruity sweetness.

* Cheesy scrambled eggs.

* Chopped fruit and yoghurt.

* And for lazier weekend mornings – pancakes with blue-berries, sliced strawberries or chopped banana set in them.

Q My two-year-old daughter refuses to eat anything but baked beans or spaghetti hoops for her lunch or tea. I try all sorts, like cottage pie, pasta, fish pie, Bolognese, but get a 'no'. Today I gave her cottage pie, she ate five

mouthfuls and then pushed the food away, so for the first time I refused to give her any pudding and she went to bed without eating anything else. I feel really guilty and unsure whether I should persevere with this tactic but I'm concerned she isn't get enough variety of food, especially vegetables.

A There aren't many more infuriating things than having a toddler spit out a lovely meal you have just slaved to make – especially when they are delighted to eat something as simple as baked beans. You are right to persevere though, for many reasons. Firstly, thinking about what a growing child needs, the meals you make are going to bring a much wider range of vital nutrients to your daughter than cans of just one or two preferred foods. Also, home-prepared food without added salt is much lower in sodium or salt. Regular canned baked beans or spaghetti hoops contain significant amounts of salt – as well as the health aspect, I feel this might also dull her palate for other foods. Lastly, it is through this persevering that your daughter is going to start eating a wider range of foods, meaning that there's less chance of her becoming a fussy eater and increasing the chance that you can all enjoy the same meal together as a family.

When you are making up a batch of meals, you could try making your own baked beans (without added salt). You'll find traditional baked bean recipes if you do a search on the Internet – they are somewhat different to the canned variety, but still very tasty for all the family. They're also lower in salt if you leave out any bacon or salted pork (like gammon) in the recipe. They were a staple of cowboys in the American West, and originated in Boston in the 1850s, so you are really exposing your child to ethnic cuisine! As a bonus, one serving of pulses (dried beans, lentils, chickpeas, etc) count as one serving of vegetables for the day. So you can use the baked beans, or lentil soup or hummus, to help your daughter reach her five a day.

To address the other issue – vegetables – start by keeping a food diary for three days. See how many servings of vegetables your daughter eats on average – look for two or three servings a day, preferably including two different colours each day, e.g. green peas and orange carrots. If she is having less than this, think about ways to include more. This could be as:

* Chopped raw veg, such as carrot sticks, mange tout and strips of peppers, with hummus dip as a snack.
* Microwaved frozen veg (perfect for busy mums).
* Grated veg such as carrots, courgette or butternut squash mixed into dishes such as pasta sauce, cottage pie or fish pie. To save time, you could also use frozen vegetables pulsed briefly with a food processor or hand-held blender.
* Soups containing puréed vegetables, such as carrot or pumpkin soup.

If you really find it impossible to persuade her to eat enough vegetables, you could discuss a balanced multivitamin supplement with your GP or health visitor.

I also think that you should take a close look at your daughter's snacking. Many children need to be truly hungry before they venture on to trying new foods and, if they have eaten just a couple of hours beforehand, they may not reach this point. I'd suggest starting by halving the size of her snacks. If that doesn't work, you could cut down further, or even try just giving her a drink at snack-time to put something in her tummy. You could also try putting a very small amount of baked beans or spaghetti hoops on her plate to start her off, and hopefully she'll move on to other foods that are offered. Do look for the lower-salt types though.

Q I am having a testing time with my 17-month-old boy who weighs around 11.5kg (26lb) and is about 86cm (34in) tall. He is quickly changing from a terrific eater to a real fusspot. He will eat brilliantly at nursery but at home he pushes the spoon away. He does like feeding himself, but when I get in from work I just want something quick

and easy, otherwise it gets too late and he is really tired and irritable. Also, I was just wondering what other people's toddlers of a similar age eat and drink in a day and how much they weigh?

A Don't worry too much if your son is not really hungry after nursery. It sounds as if he eats very well during the day, possibly because it's more like a fun game to eat with the other children. While adults often eat from habit, and will eat supper just because it's suppertime, even if we're not hungry, young children naturally tend to regulate their intake to match their calorie requirements more closely. Thus, if your son has eaten a lot earlier in the day, he may not have a great appetite at night. Getting food on the table quickly can help matters at this time of day though. As you mentioned, children can get tired and grumpy in the evening, and this can make them less likely to sit and eat. If your son has already had a cooked meal at nursery, you could try tempting him with soup and toast (especially in colder weather) or a simple sandwich. If he needs something more substantial, here are a few quick and easy meal ideas to help get supper on the table earlier:

* Pasta with a commercial tomato pasta sauce (check for those with little or no salt added) and grated cheese.

* Pasta or rice with a spoon of cream cheese, protein food such as chopped chicken or tinned salmon, and vegetables including chopped tomato, tinned sweetcorn (without added salt) or frozen peas.

* Pitta bread filled with tinned tuna, chopped tomatoes and a little cheese, maybe warmed in the oven or microwave.

* Baked potato (cooked in the microwave if time is short) with beans or tuna mayonnaise, and carrot and celery sticks on the side.

* Scrambled egg with finely sliced red and green peppers added, served with toast fingers.

You can find many more delicious meal ideas for toddlers, such as Fruity Chicken Salad and Neapolitan Macaroni, in *The Gina Ford Baby and Toddler Cook Book*.

The amount toddlers eat in a day can vary widely, but at your son's age as a rule his diet would comprise three small meals and two snacks daily, including three or four portions of carbohydrate or starchy foods (bread, other grain foods and potatoes), five portions of fruit and vegetables, two portions of meat and meat alternatives, and a minimum of 350ml (12oz) and a maximum of 500ml (17oz) of full-fat milk per day or equivalent dairy foods. Do note that many energetic children will eat more than this and that appetites go up and down. Therefore, don't be concerned if your son's intake doesn't match these guidelines every day; think about it as an average intake over three or four days. Your health visitor or GP will be able to check his progress if you have any concerns about the rate he is gaining in inches or pounds. However, you can be reassured that your son's weight and height are well within normal ranges, with his height a little over the 91st percentile and his weight at about the 50th percentile.

Q My toddler has suddenly taken a real dislike to his milk and is now taking a lot less than 350ml (12oz) a day. Some nights he flatly refuses his bedtime drink. I'm worried he's not getting the right nutrition – what should I do?

A Babies and young toddlers are not capable of distinguishing the difference between hunger and thirst, so it would be wise to make sure that your toddler is not eating too much solid food at mealtimes, which would have a knock-on effect on the amount of milk he is drinking. For several days, keep a note of all the food, milk and other fluids that he consumes over each 24-hour period and the time he consumes them. If he is eating in excess of the guidelines for his age, try cutting back on the solids he consumes and see if this helps increase the milk he will take in.

When toddlers refuse milk at this age it is sometimes because they have drunk too much water or juice in the afternoon, which then affects their bedtime bottle. Try to offer your child a mid-afternoon drink of water only no later than 3pm, and offer only a couple of ounces of fluids with his tea.

If your toddler still refuses his milk, offer him a yoghurt at both breakfast and lunch and include a serving of cheese in his daily diet. Also try to include extra sauces and milk puddings in his diet, and milk-shake drinks made with fruit or fromage frais yoghurt. This will help boost his intake and ensure he gets that right balance of vitamins and minerals.

Q **My son has always been a good eater, but about four weeks ago he got a bad chesty cold. He is better now but is still not eating properly. He eats a Weetabix for breakfast, sometimes a breadstick as a morning**

snack, cheese spread sandwiches and an organic, child-sized yoghurt for lunch. I offer him a proper meal every teatime, but every night it is refused. Until yesterday he has been having a little cup of milk when he wakes from his nap, but I decided to cut that out today in an attempt to get him to eat better. How do I encourage my son to go back to eating the variety of foods he used to? He hasn't eaten any fresh fruit or vegetables now for about four weeks.

A Coaxing a child back into eating well again after illness can take time and determination, especially with children in this age group whose appetite can be small even when they are well. Now that you feel your son is much better you may have to begin to get a little firmer about offering him something else when a meal is refused. Although you were lenient during his illness, now that he has recovered you can begin not to offer alternatives if a meal is refused. Very few toddlers will starve themselves. If they are really hungry and offered tasty, attractive, small meals they will accept them once they have realised there is no option being given. It may take a few days for this to happen and your son may protest, but persistence and remaining calm about food and his intake will help you immensely.

Give him portions which are smaller than he may have had in the past and serve food in bite-sized pieces. It is far better for both of you if he clears his plate of a small portion, than picks away and appears to eat little of a larger one. Dips are often popular. You can try a simple tomato sauce recipe and offer with steamed vegetable batons as well as one or two chicken or fish goujons to dip into it.

Once he has finished the food on his plate ask him if he would like a little more, but don't push him. Give him a very small portion of 'seconds' if he would like some, and if he doesn't manage to finish it then just remove his plate.

If your son rejects a meal, then without comment take the dish away and let him get down from the table. Offering him an alternative or yoghurt is no longer an option if you want things to change. It can be hard when you worry that your child is not eating but by not offering an alternative he will soon start to accept your meals again.

If your son normally has a snack mid-morning or mid-afternoon, wait until then to offer him something else to eat. Try to make sure that this snack time is at least two hours before his next meal is due. Again you should try and entice him to accept different foods, even though you may want to give him the things you know he will take, such as bread-sticks. To help him get used to fruit again make up some ice lollies using fresh juice or natural yoghurt flavoured with fruit purée and frozen. Another idea would be to have a selection of different fruits and use them as batons for a natural yoghurt dip. Again keep the portions very small, and take time to enjoy sharing a snack like this with your son. Don't push him to eat more than he wants. Remove the snack after 15–20 minutes and try not to comment if he has eaten nothing. Praise him when he does try something, but remaining calm and matter of fact about the whole issue is the best approach.

Keep a diary of what he eats each day, however small it appears to you. Looking at the overview of a week you will probably find he has begun to eat a wider variety of food again, once sandwiches and toast are no longer always offered. His appetite may still be small, as it can take a while for a toddler to regain this after a time of illness.

If, after a week of serving small, attractive meals with no alternatives, your son is still refusing to eat properly it would be wise to discuss your concerns with your health visitor or GP.

Q **I have a little boy, who will turn two next month. Over the past few weeks I've been getting concerned that he's not eating enough. He used to guzzle every meal, no matter what was offered, but now he just picks at some meals and I can't seem to do anything to make him finish what's on the plate.**

A Just as you can lead a horse to water but can't make them drink, there is sometimes nothing you can do to get your toddler to eat his meal. But this is generally no cause for concern. Virtually all children naturally eat enough to satisfy their needs, but it is often not spread evenly between the three meals of each day. They may pick at breakfast and lunch, and then demolish several platefuls at the evening meal. Or they may eat like a sparrow for a full day but make up for it with super-sized portions the next day. To reassure yourself you could try keeping a three-day food diary to examine your child's meal pattern – you just can't rely on looking at what they eat at one meal or even over one day. Note down all that is eaten over a three-day period, then add up how many portions he has eaten from each food group: dairy; meat, fish, poultry and alternatives; fruit and vegetables; and carbohydrates or starchy foods. Divide this by three to get an average amount per day and then look at your son's overall intake. You can check up on what makes up a portion and how many are recommended for each food group using

The Contented Child's Food Bible. Another tip is to check that your son isn't drinking more than the recommended amount of milk, or any more than small amounts of sweetened drinks (including fruit juices), as these can fill children up and take away their appetite for solid foods. If you would like extra reassurance you could also take your son to his health visitor or GP for a height and weight check.

You may wonder why your growing son seems to be eating less and yet remains quite healthy. Children naturally reduce their food intake relative to their body weight (in other words, they need fewer calories per kilogram of body weight) as they age, and this is most obvious during a child's second year. This happens because a baby's rate of growth is most rapid during their first year – they approximately triple their weight during this time. This slows down dramatically to about a 25 per cent weight increase during their second year.

Conclusion

Many children become fussy eaters at some time in their lives but please be comforted by the fact that most do grow out of it, and a period of fussy eating is unlikely to cause damage to your children's eating habits in the long term.

Mealtime battles and sudden changes to a child's eating habits can be highly stressful for the whole family, with parents concerned that their toddlers are not eating enough or getting a balanced diet. The important thing is to try and stay calm, and not to force your child into eating either by nagging or offering bribes of pudding or treats. I know you may worry that he will starve if he misses a meal but trust me; he will eat when he is hungry enough. Once he realises that you are not going to make a fuss if he misses a meal and, more importantly, that he is not going to be offered alternatives or puddings or treats, he will soon learn to enjoy his food again.

I hope that the tips and advice in this book, based on my own experience of advising and working with families, and from the invaluable feedback I get from parents, will help you change your own fussy eater into a confident, healthy one.

For further advice and support, please do visit my website www.contentedtoddler.com, which has many success stories and case studies on how parents have resolved their problems of fussy feeding.

Useful Resources

Allergy UK
Helpline: 01322 619898
www.allergyuk.org

CASH (Concensus Action on Salt and Health)
Tel: 020 7882 5941
www.actiononsalt.org.uk

Food Standards Agency
Tel: 020 7276 8829
www.food.gov.uk

The Foundation for the Study of Infant Deaths (FSID)
Helpline: 0808 802 6868
www.fsid.org.uk

La Leche League
Tel: 0845 456 1855
www.laleche.org.uk

NCT (The National Childbirth Trust)
Tel: 0300 330 0770
www.nctpregnancyandbabycare.com

Soil Association
Tel: 0117 314 5000
www.soilassociation.org

Sure Start
Tel: 08002 346 346
www.direct.gov.uk/surestart

Twins and Multiple Births Association (TAMBA)
Tel: 01483 304442
Twinline: 0800 138 0509
www.tamba.org.uk

Vegetarian Society
Includes advice on a gluten-free diet.
Tel: 0161 925 2000
www.vegsoc.org/info/gluten.html

Further Reading

The New Contented Little Baby Book by Gina Ford (Vermilion 2006)

The Contented Toddler Years by Gina Ford (Vermilion 2006)

The Contented Baby with Toddler Book by Gina Ford (Vermilion 2009)

The Contented Little Baby Book of Weaning by Gina Ford (Vermilion 2006)

The Complete Sleep Guide for Contented Babies and Toddlers by Gina Ford (Vermilion 2006)

The Contented Baby's First Year by Gina Ford (Vermilion 2007)

Potty Training in One Week by Gina Ford (Vermilion 2003)

A Contented House with Twins by Gina Ford and Alice Beer (Vermilion 2006)

The Gina Ford Baby and Toddler Cook Book by Gina Ford (Vermilion 2005)

Feeding Made Easy by Gina Ford (Vermilion 2008)

The Contented Child's Food Bible by Gina Ford (Vermilion 2005)

Gina Ford's Top Tips for Contented Babies and Toddlers by Gina Ford (Vermilion 2006)

From Crying Baby to Contented Baby by Gina Ford (Vermilion 2010)

Contented Baby Newsletter

To learn more about the Contented Baby routines and Gina Ford's books visit Gina's official websites at www.contentedbaby.com and www.contentedtoddler.com and sign up to receive Gina's free monthly newsletter, which is full of useful information, tips and advice as well as answers to questions about parenting issues and even a recipe or two.

You may also want to become part of Gina's online community by joining one or both of the websites. As a member you'll receive a monthly online magazine with a personal message from Gina, along with a selection of the latest exclusive features on topical issues from our guest contributors and members. You'll be able to access more than 2,000 frequently asked questions about feeding, sleeping and development answered by Gina and her team, as well as many case histories not featured in the Contented Little Baby series of books.

www.contentedbaby.com
www.contentedtoddler.com

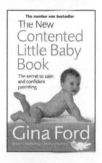

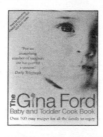

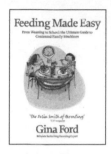